I0448003

My Personal Diet and Weight Loss Log

by Ellen Thorne Publishing

Acknowledgement:

Front cover photo image source: Alan Cleaver, reproduced under Wikimedia Commons license.

Introduction

Maintaining a healthy and desirable weight is a constant struggle for most people. It is not unusual to put on an additional 10 or 20 pounds, or even more, particularly as we age. Many diets and exercise programs have been developed over the years, but it is our belief that the easiest way to understand weight loss and reach long term results is still by counting calories. But to even begin realizing success, you must first have a good understanding of how many calories you consume in a typical day, and how many you need to cut in order to lose even one pound of weight.

First, you burn calories even when sleeping, on the average around 60 per hour. This means that even if you don't exercise at all, you'll still burn around 1400 calories per day, give or take a couple of hundred depending on your weight (heavier people burn slightly more than lighter weight people).

Second, you must know how many calories you need to consume throughout a typical day in order to keep your weight constant, so you must consider not only your weight, but also how active you are in your daily routine. You can easily find calorie calculators online that will help you with this estimation. As a guideline, most people will need somewhere between 1,700 and 2,500 calories per day.

Third, in order to lose even one pound of weight, you must know how many calories this pound contains. One pound of fat contains approximately 3,500 calories.

As an example, let's say that you are a 150-pound female desiring to weigh 135 pounds. You are moderately active and have remained steady at 150 pounds for some time. You will now calculate the number of calories you consume in a typical day. You can easily find this information on just about all packaged food, and also on many restaurant menus. But you must be brutally honest and ensure that you calculate the calories correctly. When reading the information on the food packaging, make sure you understand exactly how much a "serving" is.

For a comfortable weight loss of one pound per week, you'll need to cut 500 calories per day from your typical daily diet. (500 calories X 7 days = 3,500 calories, which is equal to one pound of weight loss per week.) At this rate, it would take you fifteen weeks, or roughly four months to lose 15 pounds, and reach your ideal weight of 135 pounds.

Losing one pound per week is not a quick weight loss, but it is a very manageable weight loss that just anybody with the right motivation can succeed with. If you want to lose weight quicker, you must cut more calories from your diet. You can also exercise more; however, keep in mind that to lose even one pound of weight through exercise, the average person must walk a distance of approximately 35 miles. It's far easier to lose weight through diet than through exercise.

One of the easiest ways to start losing weight is to cut sugared drinks. If you are a consumer of such, either switch to diet sodas or cut sodas and other sugared drinks entirely. One can of regular soda typically contains more than a hundred calories. So if you drink three cans a day, you can easily cut three to four hundred calories a day just by switching to diet drinks, and without changing anything else in your diet. Alcohol also contains plenty of calories, as do fruit juices. Although fruit juices are more nutritious than either alcohol or soda, they still contain a significant amount of calories, and you can't lose weight unless you cut your daily caloric intake. Another good way to start is to cut the typical size of your meals by one-fourth to one-third. If you eat three pieces of toast in the morning, cut down and eat only two. If you eat one bowl of cereal, cut down and eat only two-thirds bowl.

This journal, then, will help you keep an honest log of what you eat each day and how many calories you consume, and will thus start you on the path to a healthy weight loss program that you can live with for the long haul. On the next page, start by recording your current weight and your weight loss goal, how many calories you typically consume in one day, and how many you need to cut each day in order to reach your goal. Note that your weight will vary naturally by a few pounds from day to day and from morning to evening, depending on how much water your body retains. Then use each subsequent page to record what you eat throughout the day and how many calories each item contains. Remember that you must be brutally honest in order to get an accurate record of your progress.

Don't get discouraged if you seem to stagnate for a week now and then. Your body needs time to make the necessary adjustments, and since several factors affect your weight from day to day, it is hardly ever possible to get an accurate account of your weight on a daily basis. While some experts recommend weighing yourself only once a week, we recommend buying an accurate digital scale and weighing yourself every morning, while remaining aware that your weight will naturally fluctuate somewhat from day to day.

Best of luck!

Initial Weight Loss Assessment:

I currently weigh _____ pounds.

I typically consume _____ calories per day.

I want to lose_____ pounds by_____.

In order to meet this goal, I must cut_____ calories per day from my diet.

My daily diet will include no more than _____ calories.

Date: | Weight:

Include Food and Drink Here | Note Calories Here

Breakfast

_____ | _____
_____ | _____
_____ | _____

Lunch

_____ | _____
_____ | _____
_____ | _____

Dinner

_____ | _____
_____ | _____
_____ | _____

Snacks

_____ | _____
_____ | _____
_____ | _____

Goal Met: Yes   No | Total Calories:

Date: | Weight:

Include Food and Drink Here | Note Calories Here

Breakfast

Lunch

Dinner

Snacks

Goal Met: Yes   No | Total Calories:

Date:	Weight:

Include Food and Drink Here | Note Calories Here

Breakfast

Lunch

Dinner

Snacks

Goal Met: Yes   No | Total Calories:

Date: | Weight:

Include Food and Drink Here | Note Calories Here

Breakfast

_____ | _____
_____ | _____
_____ | _____
_____ | _____

Lunch

_____ | _____
_____ | _____
_____ | _____
_____ | _____

Dinner

_____ | _____
_____ | _____
_____ | _____
_____ | _____

Snacks

_____ | _____
_____ | _____
_____ | _____
_____ | _____

Goal Met: Yes   No | Total Calories:

Date: | Weight:

Include Food and Drink Here | Note Calories Here

Breakfast

Lunch

Dinner

Snacks

Goal Met: Yes   No | Total Calories:

Date:	Weight:
Include Food and Drink Here	Note Calories Here
Breakfast	
Lunch	
Dinner	
Snacks	
Goal Met: Yes No	Total Calories:

Date:	Weight:
Include Food and Drink Here	Note Calories Here
Breakfast	
Lunch	
Dinner	
Snacks	
Goal Met: Yes No	Total Calories:

Date:	Weight:
Include Food and Drink Here	Note Calories Here
Breakfast	
Lunch	
Dinner	
Snacks	
Goal Met: Yes No	Total Calories:

Date: _____ | Weight: _____

Include Food and Drink Here | Note Calories Here

Breakfast

_____ | _____
_____ | _____
_____ | _____

Lunch

_____ | _____
_____ | _____
_____ | _____

Dinner

_____ | _____
_____ | _____
_____ | _____

Snacks

_____ | _____
_____ | _____
_____ | _____

Goal Met: Yes   No | Total Calories:

Date:	Weight:
Include Food and Drink Here	Note Calories Here
Breakfast	
Lunch	
Dinner	
Snacks	
Goal Met: Yes No	Total Calories:

Date:	Weight:
Include Food and Drink Here	Note Calories Here
Breakfast	
Lunch	
Dinner	
Snacks	
Goal Met: Yes No	Total Calories:

Date:	Weight:
Include Food and Drink Here	Note Calories Here
Breakfast	
Lunch	
Dinner	
Snacks	
Goal Met: Yes No	Total Calories:

Date:	Weight:
Include Food and Drink Here	Note Calories Here
Breakfast	
Lunch	
Dinner	
Snacks	
Goal Met: Yes No	Total Calories:

Date: | Weight:

Include Food and Drink Here | Note Calories Here

Breakfast

_____

_____

_____

_____

Lunch

_____

_____

_____

_____

Dinner

_____

_____

_____

_____

Snacks

_____

_____

_____

_____

Goal Met: Yes   No | Total Calories:

Date:	Weight:
Include Food and Drink Here	Note Calories Here
Breakfast	
Lunch	
Dinner	
Snacks	
Goal Met: Yes No	Total Calories:

Date:	Weight:
Include Food and Drink Here	Note Calories Here
Breakfast	
Lunch	
Dinner	
Snacks	
Goal Met: Yes No	Total Calories:

Date:	Weight:
Include Food and Drink Here	Note Calories Here
Breakfast	
Lunch	
Dinner	
Snacks	
Goal Met: Yes No	Total Calories:

Date:	Weight:
Include Food and Drink Here	Note Calories Here
Breakfast	
Lunch	
Dinner	
Snacks	
Goal Met: Yes No	Total Calories:

Date:	Weight:
Include Food and Drink Here	Note Calories Here
Breakfast	
Lunch	
Dinner	
Snacks	
Goal Met: Yes No	Total Calories:

Date:	Weight:
Include Food and Drink Here	Note Calories Here
Breakfast	
Lunch	
Dinner	
Snacks	
Goal Met: Yes No	Total Calories:

Date:	Weight:

Include Food and Drink Here | Note Calories Here

Breakfast

_____ | _____
_____ | _____
_____ | _____
_____ | _____

Lunch

_____ | _____
_____ | _____
_____ | _____
_____ | _____

Dinner

_____ | _____
_____ | _____
_____ | _____
_____ | _____

Snacks

_____ | _____
_____ | _____
_____ | _____
_____ | _____

Goal Met: Yes   No | Total Calories:

Date:	Weight:
Include Food and Drink Here	Note Calories Here
Breakfast	
Lunch	
Dinner	
Snacks	
Goal Met: Yes No	Total Calories:

Date:	Weight:
Include Food and Drink Here	Note Calories Here
Breakfast	
Lunch	
Dinner	
Snacks	
Goal Met: Yes No	Total Calories:

Date: | Weight:

Include Food and Drink Here | Note Calories Here

Breakfast

_____ | _____
_____ | _____
_____ | _____
_____ | _____

Lunch

_____ | _____
_____ | _____
_____ | _____
_____ | _____

Dinner

_____ | _____
_____ | _____
_____ | _____
_____ | _____

Snacks

_____ | _____
_____ | _____
_____ | _____
_____ | _____

Goal Met: Yes   No | Total Calories:

Date: | Weight:

Include Food and Drink Here | Note Calories Here

Breakfast

_____ | _____
_____ | _____
_____ | _____
_____ | _____

Lunch

_____ | _____
_____ | _____
_____ | _____

Dinner

_____ | _____
_____ | _____
_____ | _____
_____ | _____

Snacks

_____ | _____
_____ | _____
_____ | _____

Goal Met: Yes   No | Total Calories:

Date:	Weight:
Include Food and Drink Here	Note Calories Here
Breakfast	
Lunch	
Dinner	
Snacks	
Goal Met: Yes No	Total Calories:

Date: | Weight:

Include Food and Drink Here | Note Calories Here

Breakfast

_____ | _____
_____ | _____
_____ | _____
_____ | _____

Lunch

_____ | _____
_____ | _____
_____ | _____
_____ | _____

Dinner

_____ | _____
_____ | _____
_____ | _____
_____ | _____

Snacks

_____ | _____
_____ | _____
_____ | _____
_____ | _____

Goal Met: Yes   No | Total Calories:

Date:	Weight:
Include Food and Drink Here	Note Calories Here
Breakfast	
Lunch	
Dinner	
Snacks	
Goal Met: Yes No	Total Calories:

Date:	Weight:
Include Food and Drink Here	Note Calories Here
Breakfast	
Lunch	
Dinner	
Snacks	
Goal Met: Yes No	Total Calories:

Date:	Weight:
Include Food and Drink Here	Note Calories Here
Breakfast	
Lunch	
Dinner	
Snacks	
Goal Met: Yes No	Total Calories:

Date:	Weight:
Include Food and Drink Here	Note Calories Here
Breakfast	
Lunch	
Dinner	
Snacks	
Goal Met: Yes No	Total Calories:

Date:	Weight:
Include Food and Drink Here	Note Calories Here
Breakfast	
Lunch	
Dinner	
Snacks	
Goal Met: Yes No	Total Calories:

Date:	Weight:
Include Food and Drink Here	Note Calories Here
Breakfast	
Lunch	
Dinner	
Snacks	
Goal Met: Yes No	Total Calories:

Date: | Weight:

Include Food and Drink Here | Note Calories Here

Breakfast

_____

_____

_____

_____

Lunch

_____

_____

_____

_____

Dinner

_____

_____

_____

_____

Snacks

_____

_____

_____

_____

Goal Met: Yes   No | Total Calories:

Date: | Weight:

Include Food and Drink Here | Note Calories Here

Breakfast

Lunch

Dinner

Snacks

Goal Met: Yes   No | Total Calories:

Date:	Weight:
Include Food and Drink Here	Note Calories Here
Breakfast	
Lunch	
Dinner	
Snacks	
Goal Met: Yes No	Total Calories:

Date:	Weight:
Include Food and Drink Here	Note Calories Here
Breakfast	
Lunch	
Dinner	
Snacks	
Goal Met: Yes No	Total Calories:

Date: | Weight:

Include Food and Drink Here | Note Calories Here

Breakfast

_____ | _____
_____ | _____
_____ | _____

Lunch

_____ | _____
_____ | _____
_____ | _____

Dinner

_____ | _____
_____ | _____
_____ | _____

Snacks

_____ | _____
_____ | _____
_____ | _____

Goal Met: Yes   No | Total Calories:

Date: | Weight:

Include Food and Drink Here | Note Calories Here

Breakfast

Lunch

Dinner

Snacks

Goal Met: Yes   No | Total Calories:

Date: | Weight:

Include Food and Drink Here | Note Calories Here

Breakfast

Lunch

Dinner

Snacks

Goal Met: Yes   No | Total Calories:

Date: | Weight:

Include Food and Drink Here | Note Calories Here

Breakfast

Lunch

Dinner

Snacks

Goal Met: Yes   No | Total Calories:

Date: | Weight:

Include Food and Drink Here | Note Calories Here

Breakfast

_____ | _____
_____ | _____
_____ | _____
_____ | _____

Lunch

_____ | _____
_____ | _____
_____ | _____
_____ | _____

Dinner

_____ | _____
_____ | _____
_____ | _____
_____ | _____

Snacks

_____ | _____
_____ | _____
_____ | _____
_____ | _____

Goal Met: Yes   No | Total Calories:

Date:	Weight:
Include Food and Drink Here	Note Calories Here
Breakfast	
Lunch	
Dinner	
Snacks	
Goal Met: Yes No	Total Calories:

Date: | Weight:

Include Food and Drink Here | Note Calories Here

Breakfast

Lunch

Dinner

Snacks

Goal Met: Yes   No | Total Calories:

Date:	Weight:
Include Food and Drink Here	Note Calories Here
Breakfast	
Lunch	
Dinner	
Snacks	
Goal Met: Yes No	Total Calories:

Date:	Weight:
Include Food and Drink Here	Note Calories Here
Breakfast	
Lunch	
Dinner	
Snacks	
Goal Met: Yes No	Total Calories:

Date: Weight:

Include Food and Drink Here   Note Calories Here

Breakfast

Lunch

Dinner

Snacks

Goal Met: Yes   No   Total Calories:

Date:	Weight:
Include Food and Drink Here	Note Calories Here
Breakfast	
Lunch	
Dinner	
Snacks	
Goal Met: Yes No	Total Calories:

Date: | Weight:

Include Food and Drink Here | Note Calories Here

Breakfast

Lunch

Dinner

Snacks

Goal Met: Yes   No | Total Calories:

Date:	Weight:
Include Food and Drink Here	Note Calories Here
Breakfast	
Lunch	
Dinner	
Snacks	
Goal Met: Yes No	Total Calories:

Date:	Weight:
Include Food and Drink Here	Note Calories Here
Breakfast	
Lunch	
Dinner	
Snacks	
Goal Met: Yes No	Total Calories:

Date:	Weight:
Include Food and Drink Here	Note Calories Here
Breakfast	
Lunch	
Dinner	
Snacks	
Goal Met: Yes No	Total Calories:

Date:	Weight:
Include Food and Drink Here	Note Calories Here
Breakfast	
Lunch	
Dinner	
Snacks	
Goal Met: Yes No	Total Calories:

Date:	Weight:
Include Food and Drink Here	Note Calories Here
Breakfast	
Lunch	
Dinner	
Snacks	
Goal Met: Yes No	Total Calories:

Date: | Weight:

Include Food and Drink Here | Note Calories Here

Breakfast

Lunch

Dinner

Snacks

Goal Met: Yes   No | Total Calories:

Date:	Weight:
Include Food and Drink Here	Note Calories Here
Breakfast	
Lunch	
Dinner	
Snacks	
Goal Met: Yes No	Total Calories:

Date: | Weight:

Include Food and Drink Here | Note Calories Here

Breakfast

Lunch

Dinner

Snacks

Goal Met: Yes   No | Total Calories:

Date:	Weight:
Include Food and Drink Here	Note Calories Here
Breakfast	
Lunch	
Dinner	
Snacks	
Goal Met: Yes No	Total Calories:

Date: | Weight:

Include Food and Drink Here | Note Calories Here

Breakfast

_____

_____

_____

Lunch

_____

_____

_____

Dinner

_____

_____

_____

Snacks

_____

_____

_____

Goal Met: Yes   No | Total Calories:

Date: | Weight:

Include Food and Drink Here | Note Calories Here

Breakfast

_____ | _____

_____ | _____

_____ | _____

Lunch

_____ | _____

_____ | _____

_____ | _____

Dinner

_____ | _____

_____ | _____

_____ | _____

Snacks

_____ | _____

_____ | _____

_____ | _____

Goal Met: Yes   No | Total Calories:

Date:	Weight:
Include Food and Drink Here	Note Calories Here
Breakfast	
Lunch	
Dinner	
Snacks	
Goal Met: Yes No	Total Calories:

Date: | Weight:

Include Food and Drink Here | Note Calories Here

Breakfast

_____

_____

_____

Lunch

_____

_____

_____

Dinner

_____

_____

_____

Snacks

_____

_____

_____

Goal Met: Yes   No | Total Calories:

Date: | Weight:

Include Food and Drink Here | Note Calories Here

Breakfast

Lunch

Dinner

Snacks

Goal Met: Yes   No | Total Calories:

Date: | Weight:

Include Food and Drink Here | Note Calories Here

Breakfast

Lunch

Dinner

Snacks

Goal Met: Yes   No | Total Calories:

Date:	Weight:
Include Food and Drink Here	Note Calories Here
Breakfast	
Lunch	
Dinner	
Snacks	
Goal Met: Yes No	Total Calories:

Date: | Weight:

Include Food and Drink Here | Note Calories Here

Breakfast

Lunch

Dinner

Snacks

Goal Met: Yes   No | Total Calories:

Date:	Weight:
Include Food and Drink Here	Note Calories Here
Breakfast	
Lunch	
Dinner	
Snacks	
Goal Met: Yes No	Total Calories:

Date: | Weight:

Include Food and Drink Here | Note Calories Here

Breakfast

_____ | _____
_____ | _____
_____ | _____
_____ | _____

Lunch

_____ | _____
_____ | _____
_____ | _____
_____ | _____

Dinner

_____ | _____
_____ | _____
_____ | _____
_____ | _____

Snacks

_____ | _____
_____ | _____
_____ | _____
_____ | _____

Goal Met: Yes   No | Total Calories:

Date:	Weight:
Include Food and Drink Here	Note Calories Here
Breakfast	
Lunch	
Dinner	
Snacks	
Goal Met: Yes No	Total Calories:

Date: | Weight:

Include Food and Drink Here | Note Calories Here

Breakfast

Lunch

Dinner

Snacks

Goal Met: Yes   No | Total Calories:

Date: | Weight:

Include Food and Drink Here | Note Calories Here

Breakfast

_____

_____

_____

_____

Lunch

_____

_____

_____

_____

Dinner

_____

_____

_____

_____

Snacks

_____

_____

_____

_____

Goal Met: Yes   No | Total Calories:

Date: | Weight:

Include Food and Drink Here | Note Calories Here

Breakfast

Lunch

Dinner

Snacks

Goal Met: Yes   No | Total Calories:

Date:	Weight:
Include Food and Drink Here	Note Calories Here
Breakfast	
Lunch	
Dinner	
Snacks	
Goal Met: Yes No	Total Calories:

Date: | Weight:

Include Food and Drink Here | Note Calories Here

Breakfast

_____ | _____
_____ | _____
_____ | _____

Lunch

_____ | _____
_____ | _____
_____ | _____

Dinner

_____ | _____
_____ | _____
_____ | _____

Snacks

_____ | _____
_____ | _____
_____ | _____

Goal Met: Yes   No | Total Calories:

Date:	Weight:
Include Food and Drink Here	Note Calories Here
Breakfast	
Lunch	
Dinner	
Snacks	
Goal Met: Yes No	Total Calories:

Date: | Weight:

Include Food and Drink Here | Note Calories Here

Breakfast

_____ | _____
_____ | _____
_____ | _____
_____ | _____

Lunch

_____ | _____
_____ | _____
_____ | _____
_____ | _____

Dinner

_____ | _____
_____ | _____
_____ | _____
_____ | _____

Snacks

_____ | _____
_____ | _____
_____ | _____
_____ | _____

Goal Met: Yes   No | Total Calories:

Date: | Weight:

Include Food and Drink Here | Note Calories Here

Breakfast

_____ | _____
_____ | _____
_____ | _____

Lunch

_____ | _____
_____ | _____
_____ | _____

Dinner

_____ | _____
_____ | _____
_____ | _____

Snacks

_____ | _____
_____ | _____
_____ | _____

Goal Met: Yes   No | Total Calories:

Date:	Weight:
Include Food and Drink Here	Note Calories Here
Breakfast	
Lunch	
Dinner	
Snacks	
Goal Met: Yes No	Total Calories:

Date: | Weight:

Include Food and Drink Here | Note Calories Here

Breakfast

Lunch

Dinner

Snacks

Goal Met: Yes   No | Total Calories:

Date: | Weight:

Include Food and Drink Here | Note Calories Here

Breakfast

Lunch

Dinner

Snacks

Goal Met: Yes   No | Total Calories:

Date:	Weight:
Include Food and Drink Here	Note Calories Here
Breakfast	
Lunch	
Dinner	
Snacks	
Goal Met: Yes No	Total Calories:

Date:	Weight:
Include Food and Drink Here	Note Calories Here
Breakfast	
Lunch	
Dinner	
Snacks	
Goal Met: Yes No	Total Calories:

Date: _____ | Weight: _____

Include Food and Drink Here | Note Calories Here

Breakfast

_____ | _____

_____ | _____

_____ | _____

Lunch

_____ | _____

_____ | _____

_____ | _____

Dinner

_____ | _____

_____ | _____

_____ | _____

Snacks

_____ | _____

_____ | _____

_____ | _____

Goal Met: Yes   No | Total Calories:

Date: | Weight:

Include Food and Drink Here | Note Calories Here

Breakfast

Lunch

Dinner

Snacks

Goal Met: Yes   No | Total Calories:

Date: | Weight:

Include Food and Drink Here | Note Calories Here

Breakfast

Lunch

Dinner

Snacks

Goal Met: Yes   No | Total Calories:

Date: | Weight:

Include Food and Drink Here | Note Calories Here

Breakfast

_____ | _____
_____ | _____
_____ | _____
_____ | _____

Lunch

_____ | _____
_____ | _____
_____ | _____
_____ | _____

Dinner

_____ | _____
_____ | _____
_____ | _____
_____ | _____

Snacks

_____ | _____
_____ | _____
_____ | _____
_____ | _____

Goal Met: Yes   No | Total Calories:

Date:	Weight:
Include Food and Drink Here	Note Calories Here
Breakfast	
Lunch	
Dinner	
Snacks	
Goal Met: Yes No	Total Calories:

Date:	Weight:
Include Food and Drink Here	Note Calories Here

Breakfast

Lunch

Dinner

Snacks

Goal Met: Yes   No

Total Calories:

Date:	Weight:
Include Food and Drink Here	Note Calories Here
Breakfast	
Lunch	
Dinner	
Snacks	
Goal Met: Yes No	Total Calories:

Date: | Weight:

Include Food and Drink Here | Note Calories Here

Breakfast

_____

Lunch

_____

Dinner

_____

Snacks

_____

Goal Met: Yes   No | Total Calories:

Date:	Weight:
Include Food and Drink Here	Note Calories Here
Breakfast	
Lunch	
Dinner	
Snacks	
Goal Met: Yes No	Total Calories:

Date: | Weight:

Include Food and Drink Here | Note Calories Here

Breakfast

_____ | _____
_____ | _____
_____ | _____
_____ | _____

Lunch

_____ | _____
_____ | _____
_____ | _____
_____ | _____

Dinner

_____ | _____
_____ | _____
_____ | _____
_____ | _____

Snacks

_____ | _____
_____ | _____
_____ | _____
_____ | _____

Goal Met: Yes   No | Total Calories:

Date:	Weight:
Include Food and Drink Here	Note Calories Here
Breakfast	
Lunch	
Dinner	
Snacks	
Goal Met: Yes No	Total Calories:

Date:	Weight:
Include Food and Drink Here	Note Calories Here
Breakfast	
Lunch	
Dinner	
Snacks	
Goal Met: Yes No	Total Calories:

Date: | Weight:

Include Food and Drink Here | Note Calories Here

Breakfast

Lunch

Dinner

Snacks

Goal Met: Yes   No | Total Calories:

Date:	Weight:
Include Food and Drink Here	Note Calories Here
Breakfast	
Lunch	
Dinner	
Snacks	
Goal Met: Yes No	Total Calories:

Date: | Weight:

Include Food and Drink Here | Note Calories Here

Breakfast

Lunch

Dinner

Snacks

Goal Met: Yes   No | Total Calories:

Date:	Weight:
Include Food and Drink Here	Note Calories Here
Breakfast	
Lunch	
Dinner	
Snacks	
Goal Met: Yes No	Total Calories:

Date:	Weight:
Include Food and Drink Here	Note Calories Here
Breakfast	
Lunch	
Dinner	
Snacks	
Goal Met: Yes No	Total Calories:

Date: | Weight:

Include Food and Drink Here | Note Calories Here

Breakfast

Lunch

Dinner

Snacks

Goal Met: Yes   No | Total Calories:

Date:	Weight:
Include Food and Drink Here	Note Calories Here
Breakfast	
Lunch	
Dinner	
Snacks	
Goal Met: Yes No	Total Calories:

Date:	Weight:
Include Food and Drink Here	Note Calories Here
Breakfast	
Lunch	
Dinner	
Snacks	
Goal Met: Yes No	Total Calories:

Date:	Weight:
Include Food and Drink Here	Note Calories Here
Breakfast	
Lunch	
Dinner	
Snacks	
Goal Met: Yes No	Total Calories:

Date:	Weight:
Include Food and Drink Here	Note Calories Here

Breakfast

Lunch

Dinner

Snacks

| Goal Met: Yes   No | Total Calories: |

Date: | Weight:

Include Food and Drink Here | Note Calories Here

Breakfast

Lunch

Dinner

Snacks

Goal Met: Yes   No | Total Calories:

Date:	Weight:
Include Food and Drink Here	Note Calories Here
Breakfast	
Lunch	
Dinner	
Snacks	
Goal Met: Yes No	Total Calories:

Date:	Weight:
Include Food and Drink Here	Note Calories Here
Breakfast	
Lunch	
Dinner	
Snacks	
Goal Met: Yes No	Total Calories:

Date: | Weight:

Include Food and Drink Here | Note Calories Here

Breakfast

_____

_____

_____

_____

Lunch

_____

_____

_____

_____

Dinner

_____

_____

_____

_____

Snacks

_____

_____

_____

_____

Goal Met: Yes   No | Total Calories:

Date:	Weight:
Include Food and Drink Here	Note Calories Here
Breakfast	
Lunch	
Dinner	
Snacks	
Goal Met: Yes No	Total Calories:

Date: | Weight:

Include Food and Drink Here | Note Calories Here

Breakfast

_____

_____

_____

Lunch

_____

_____

_____

Dinner

_____

_____

_____

Snacks

_____

_____

_____

Goal Met: Yes   No | Total Calories:

Date:	Weight:
Include Food and Drink Here	Note Calories Here
Breakfast	
Lunch	
Dinner	
Snacks	
Goal Met: Yes No	Total Calories:

Date:	Weight:
Include Food and Drink Here	Note Calories Here
Breakfast	
Lunch	
Dinner	
Snacks	
Goal Met: Yes No	Total Calories:

Date:	Weight:
Include Food and Drink Here	Note Calories Here
Breakfast	
Lunch	
Dinner	
Snacks	
Goal Met: Yes No	Total Calories:

Date: | Weight:

Include Food and Drink Here | Note Calories Here

Breakfast

_____

_____

_____

Lunch

_____

_____

_____

Dinner

_____

_____

_____

Snacks

_____

_____

_____

Goal Met: Yes   No | Total Calories:

Date:	Weight:
Include Food and Drink Here	Note Calories Here
Breakfast	
Lunch	
Dinner	
Snacks	
Goal Met: Yes No	Total Calories:

Date: | Weight:

Include Food and Drink Here | Note Calories Here

Breakfast

_____ | _____

_____ | _____

_____ | _____

_____ | _____

Lunch

_____ | _____

_____ | _____

_____ | _____

_____ | _____

Dinner

_____ | _____

_____ | _____

_____ | _____

_____ | _____

Snacks

_____ | _____

_____ | _____

_____ | _____

_____ | _____

Goal Met: Yes   No | Total Calories:

Date:	Weight:
Include Food and Drink Here	Note Calories Here
Breakfast	
Lunch	
Dinner	
Snacks	
Goal Met: Yes No	Total Calories:

Date: | Weight:

Include Food and Drink Here | Note Calories Here

Breakfast

_____ | _____
_____ | _____
_____ | _____

Lunch

_____ | _____
_____ | _____
_____ | _____

Dinner

_____ | _____
_____ | _____
_____ | _____

Snacks

_____ | _____
_____ | _____
_____ | _____

Goal Met: Yes   No | Total Calories:

Date: | Weight:

Include Food and Drink Here | Note Calories Here

Breakfast

Lunch

Dinner

Snacks

Goal Met: Yes   No | Total Calories:

Date: _____ | Weight: _____

Include Food and Drink Here | Note Calories Here

Breakfast

_____ | _____
_____ | _____
_____ | _____
_____ | _____

Lunch

_____ | _____
_____ | _____
_____ | _____
_____ | _____

Dinner

_____ | _____
_____ | _____
_____ | _____
_____ | _____

Snacks

_____ | _____
_____ | _____
_____ | _____
_____ | _____

Goal Met: Yes   No | Total Calories:

Date:	Weight:
Include Food and Drink Here	Note Calories Here
Breakfast	
Lunch	
Dinner	
Snacks	
Goal Met: Yes No	Total Calories:

Date: | Weight:

Include Food and Drink Here | Note Calories Here

Breakfast

_____

_____

_____

_____

Lunch

_____

_____

_____

_____

Dinner

_____

_____

_____

_____

Snacks

_____

_____

_____

_____

Goal Met: Yes   No | Total Calories:

Date: | Weight:

Include Food and Drink Here | Note Calories Here

Breakfast

Lunch

Dinner

Snacks

Goal Met: Yes   No | Total Calories:

Date:	Weight:
Include Food and Drink Here	Note Calories Here
Breakfast	
Lunch	
Dinner	
Snacks	
Goal Met: Yes No	Total Calories:

Date:	Weight:
Include Food and Drink Here	Note Calories Here
Breakfast	
Lunch	
Dinner	
Snacks	
Goal Met: Yes No	Total Calories:

Date:	Weight:
Include Food and Drink Here	Note Calories Here
Breakfast	
Lunch	
Dinner	
Snacks	
Goal Met: Yes No	Total Calories:

Date: | Weight:

Include Food and Drink Here | Note Calories Here

Breakfast

Lunch

Dinner

Snacks

Goal Met: Yes   No | Total Calories:

Date:	Weight:
Include Food and Drink Here	Note Calories Here
Breakfast	
Lunch	
Dinner	
Snacks	
Goal Met: Yes No	Total Calories:

Date:	Weight:
Include Food and Drink Here	Note Calories Here
Breakfast	
Lunch	
Dinner	
Snacks	
Goal Met: Yes No	Total Calories:

Date:	Weight:
Include Food and Drink Here	Note Calories Here
Breakfast	
Lunch	
Dinner	
Snacks	
Goal Met: Yes No	Total Calories:

Date: | Weight:

Include Food and Drink Here | Note Calories Here

Breakfast

Lunch

Dinner

Snacks

Goal Met: Yes   No | Total Calories:

Date:	Weight:
Include Food and Drink Here	Note Calories Here
Breakfast	
Lunch	
Dinner	
Snacks	
Goal Met: Yes No	Total Calories:

Date: | Weight:

Include Food and Drink Here | Note Calories Here

Breakfast

_____ | _____
_____ | _____
_____ | _____

Lunch

_____ | _____
_____ | _____
_____ | _____

Dinner

_____ | _____
_____ | _____
_____ | _____

Snacks

_____ | _____
_____ | _____
_____ | _____

Goal Met: Yes   No | Total Calories:

Date:	Weight:
Include Food and Drink Here	Note Calories Here
Breakfast	
Lunch	
Dinner	
Snacks	
Goal Met: Yes No	Total Calories:

Date: | Weight:

Include Food and Drink Here | Note Calories Here

Breakfast

Lunch

Dinner

Snacks

Goal Met: Yes   No | Total Calories:

Date: _____ | Weight: _____

Include Food and Drink Here | Note Calories Here

Breakfast

_____ | _____
_____ | _____
_____ | _____
_____ | _____

Lunch

_____ | _____
_____ | _____
_____ | _____
_____ | _____

Dinner

_____ | _____
_____ | _____
_____ | _____
_____ | _____

Snacks

_____ | _____
_____ | _____
_____ | _____
_____ | _____

Goal Met: Yes   No | Total Calories:

Date:	Weight:
Include Food and Drink Here	Note Calories Here
Breakfast	
Lunch	
Dinner	
Snacks	
Goal Met: Yes No	Total Calories:

Date: | Weight:

Include Food and Drink Here | Note Calories Here

Breakfast

Lunch

Dinner

Snacks

Goal Met: Yes   No | Total Calories:

Date:	Weight:
Include Food and Drink Here	Note Calories Here
Breakfast	
Lunch	
Dinner	
Snacks	
Goal Met: Yes No	Total Calories:

Date: | Weight:

Include Food and Drink Here | Note Calories Here

Breakfast

_____ | _____
_____ | _____
_____ | _____

Lunch

_____ | _____
_____ | _____
_____ | _____

Dinner

_____ | _____
_____ | _____
_____ | _____

Snacks

_____ | _____
_____ | _____
_____ | _____

Goal Met: Yes   No | Total Calories:

Date:	Weight:
Include Food and Drink Here	Note Calories Here
Breakfast	
Lunch	
Dinner	
Snacks	
Goal Met: Yes No	Total Calories:

Date:	Weight:
Include Food and Drink Here	Note Calories Here
Breakfast	
Lunch	
Dinner	
Snacks	
Goal Met: Yes No	Total Calories:

Date:	Weight:
Include Food and Drink Here	Note Calories Here
Breakfast	
Lunch	
Dinner	
Snacks	
Goal Met: Yes No	Total Calories:

Date: | Weight:

Include Food and Drink Here | Note Calories Here

Breakfast

_____

Lunch

_____

Dinner

_____

Snacks

_____

Goal Met: Yes   No | Total Calories:

Date:	Weight:
Include Food and Drink Here	Note Calories Here
Breakfast	
Lunch	
Dinner	
Snacks	
Goal Met: Yes No	Total Calories:

Date: | Weight:

Include Food and Drink Here | Note Calories Here

Breakfast

Lunch

Dinner

Snacks

Goal Met: Yes   No | Total Calories:

Date:	Weight:
Include Food and Drink Here	Note Calories Here
Breakfast	
Lunch	
Dinner	
Snacks	
Goal Met: Yes No	Total Calories:

Date: | Weight:

Include Food and Drink Here | Note Calories Here

Breakfast

Lunch

Dinner

Snacks

Goal Met: Yes   No | Total Calories:

Date:	Weight:
Include Food and Drink Here	Note Calories Here
Breakfast	
Lunch	
Dinner	
Snacks	
Goal Met: Yes No	Total Calories:

Date: | Weight:

Include Food and Drink Here | Note Calories Here

Breakfast

Lunch

Dinner

Snacks

Goal Met: Yes   No | Total Calories:

Date:	Weight:
Include Food and Drink Here	Note Calories Here
Breakfast	
Lunch	
Dinner	
Snacks	
Goal Met: Yes No	Total Calories:

Date: | Weight:

Include Food and Drink Here | Note Calories Here

Breakfast

Lunch

Dinner

Snacks

Goal Met: Yes   No | Total Calories:

Date: | Weight:

Include Food and Drink Here | Note Calories Here

Breakfast

Lunch

Dinner

Snacks

Goal Met: Yes   No | Total Calories:

Date:	Weight:
Include Food and Drink Here	Note Calories Here
Breakfast	
Lunch	
Dinner	
Snacks	
Goal Met: Yes No	Total Calories:

Date: _____ | Weight: _____

Include Food and Drink Here | Note Calories Here

Breakfast

Lunch

Dinner

Snacks

Goal Met: Yes   No | Total Calories:

Date: | Weight:

Include Food and Drink Here | Note Calories Here

Breakfast

Lunch

Dinner

Snacks

Goal Met: Yes   No | Total Calories:

Date:	Weight:
Include Food and Drink Here	Note Calories Here
Breakfast	
Lunch	
Dinner	
Snacks	
Goal Met: Yes No	Total Calories:

Date: | Weight:

Include Food and Drink Here | Note Calories Here

Breakfast

_____ | _____
_____ | _____
_____ | _____
_____ | _____

Lunch

_____ | _____
_____ | _____
_____ | _____
_____ | _____

Dinner

_____ | _____
_____ | _____
_____ | _____
_____ | _____

Snacks

_____ | _____
_____ | _____
_____ | _____
_____ | _____

Goal Met: Yes   No | Total Calories:

Date: | Weight:

Include Food and Drink Here | Note Calories Here

Breakfast

Lunch

Dinner

Snacks

Goal Met: Yes   No | Total Calories:

Date: | Weight:

Include Food and Drink Here | Note Calories Here

Breakfast

_____

_____

_____

Lunch

_____

_____

_____

Dinner

_____

_____

_____

Snacks

_____

_____

_____

Goal Met: Yes   No | Total Calories:

Date: | Weight:

Include Food and Drink Here | Note Calories Here

Breakfast

Lunch

Dinner

Snacks

Goal Met: Yes   No | Total Calories:

Date: | Weight:

Include Food and Drink Here | Note Calories Here

Breakfast

_____ | _____
_____ | _____
_____ | _____
_____ | _____

Lunch

_____ | _____
_____ | _____
_____ | _____
_____ | _____

Dinner

_____ | _____
_____ | _____
_____ | _____
_____ | _____

Snacks

_____ | _____
_____ | _____
_____ | _____
_____ | _____

Goal Met: Yes   No | Total Calories:

Date:	Weight:
Include Food and Drink Here	Note Calories Here
Breakfast	
Lunch	
Dinner	
Snacks	
Goal Met: Yes No	Total Calories:

Date: | Weight:

Include Food and Drink Here | Note Calories Here

Breakfast

_____ | _____
_____ | _____
_____ | _____
_____ | _____

Lunch

_____ | _____
_____ | _____
_____ | _____
_____ | _____

Dinner

_____ | _____
_____ | _____
_____ | _____
_____ | _____

Snacks

_____ | _____
_____ | _____
_____ | _____
_____ | _____

Goal Met: Yes   No | Total Calories:

Date: | Weight:

Include Food and Drink Here | Note Calories Here

Breakfast

Lunch

Dinner

Snacks

Goal Met: Yes   No | Total Calories:

Date: | Weight:

Include Food and Drink Here | Note Calories Here

Breakfast

Lunch

Dinner

Snacks

Goal Met:　　Yes　　No | Total Calories:

Date: _____ | Weight: _____

Include Food and Drink Here | Note Calories Here

Breakfast

_____ | _____
_____ | _____
_____ | _____
_____ | _____

Lunch

_____ | _____
_____ | _____
_____ | _____
_____ | _____

Dinner

_____ | _____
_____ | _____
_____ | _____
_____ | _____

Snacks

_____ | _____
_____ | _____
_____ | _____
_____ | _____

Goal Met: Yes   No | Total Calories: _____

Date: | Weight:

Include Food and Drink Here | Note Calories Here

Breakfast

Lunch

Dinner

Snacks

Goal Met: Yes   No | Total Calories:

Date: | Weight:

Include Food and Drink Here | Note Calories Here

Breakfast

Lunch

Dinner

Snacks

Goal Met: Yes   No | Total Calories:

Date:	Weight:
Include Food and Drink Here	Note Calories Here
Breakfast	
Lunch	
Dinner	
Snacks	
Goal Met: Yes No	Total Calories:

Date:	Weight:
Include Food and Drink Here	Note Calories Here
Breakfast	
Lunch	
Dinner	
Snacks	
Goal Met: Yes No	Total Calories:

Date:	Weight:
Include Food and Drink Here	Note Calories Here
Breakfast	
Lunch	
Dinner	
Snacks	
Goal Met: Yes No	Total Calories:

Date: | Weight:

Include Food and Drink Here | Note Calories Here

Breakfast

Lunch

Dinner

Snacks

Goal Met: Yes   No | Total Calories:

Date: | Weight:

Include Food and Drink Here | Note Calories Here

Breakfast

_____ | _____
_____ | _____
_____ | _____

Lunch

_____ | _____
_____ | _____
_____ | _____

Dinner

_____ | _____
_____ | _____
_____ | _____

Snacks

_____ | _____
_____ | _____
_____ | _____

Goal Met: Yes   No | Total Calories:

Date:	Weight:
Include Food and Drink Here	Note Calories Here
Breakfast	
Lunch	
Dinner	
Snacks	
Goal Met: Yes No	Total Calories:

Date: | Weight:

Include Food and Drink Here | Note Calories Here

Breakfast

_____

Lunch

_____

Dinner

_____

Snacks

_____

Goal Met: Yes   No | Total Calories:

Date:	Weight:
Include Food and Drink Here	Note Calories Here
Breakfast	
Lunch	
Dinner	
Snacks	
Goal Met: Yes No	Total Calories:

Date: | Weight:

Include Food and Drink Here | Note Calories Here

Breakfast

_____ | _____

_____ | _____

_____ | _____

_____ | _____

Lunch

_____ | _____

_____ | _____

_____ | _____

Dinner

_____ | _____

_____ | _____

_____ | _____

Snacks

_____ | _____

_____ | _____

_____ | _____

Goal Met: Yes   No | Total Calories:

Date:	Weight:
Include Food and Drink Here	Note Calories Here
Breakfast	
Lunch	
Dinner	
Snacks	
Goal Met: Yes No	Total Calories:

Date: | Weight:

Include Food and Drink Here | Note Calories Here

Breakfast

Lunch

Dinner

Snacks

Goal Met: Yes   No | Total Calories:

Date:	Weight:
Include Food and Drink Here	Note Calories Here
Breakfast	
Lunch	
Dinner	
Snacks	
Goal Met: Yes No	Total Calories:

Date: | Weight:

Include Food and Drink Here | Note Calories Here

Breakfast

_____ | _____
_____ | _____
_____ | _____
_____ | _____

Lunch

_____ | _____
_____ | _____
_____ | _____
_____ | _____

Dinner

_____ | _____
_____ | _____
_____ | _____
_____ | _____

Snacks

_____ | _____
_____ | _____
_____ | _____
_____ | _____

Goal Met: Yes   No | Total Calories:

Date:	Weight:
Include Food and Drink Here	Note Calories Here
Breakfast	
Lunch	
Dinner	
Snacks	
Goal Met: Yes No	Total Calories:

Date:	Weight:
Include Food and Drink Here	Note Calories Here
Breakfast	
Lunch	
Dinner	
Snacks	
Goal Met: Yes No	Total Calories:

Date:	Weight:
Include Food and Drink Here	Note Calories Here
Breakfast	
Lunch	
Dinner	
Snacks	
Goal Met: Yes No	Total Calories:

Date:	Weight:
Include Food and Drink Here	Note Calories Here
Breakfast	
Lunch	
Dinner	
Snacks	
Goal Met:　　Yes　　No	Total Calories:

Date:	Weight:
Include Food and Drink Here	Note Calories Here
Breakfast	
Lunch	
Dinner	
Snacks	
Goal Met: Yes No	Total Calories:

Date: | Weight:

Include Food and Drink Here | Note Calories Here

Breakfast

_____ | _____
_____ | _____
_____ | _____
_____ | _____

Lunch

_____ | _____
_____ | _____
_____ | _____
_____ | _____

Dinner

_____ | _____
_____ | _____
_____ | _____
_____ | _____

Snacks

_____ | _____
_____ | _____
_____ | _____
_____ | _____

Goal Met: Yes   No | Total Calories:

Date: | Weight:

Include Food and Drink Here | Note Calories Here

Breakfast

Lunch

Dinner

Snacks

Goal Met: Yes   No | Total Calories:

Date: _____ | Weight: _____

Include Food and Drink Here | Note Calories Here

Breakfast

_____ | _____
_____ | _____
_____ | _____
_____ | _____

Lunch

_____ | _____
_____ | _____
_____ | _____
_____ | _____

Dinner

_____ | _____
_____ | _____
_____ | _____
_____ | _____

Snacks

_____ | _____
_____ | _____
_____ | _____
_____ | _____

Goal Met: Yes   No | Total Calories: _____

Date:	Weight:
Include Food and Drink Here	Note Calories Here
Breakfast	
Lunch	
Dinner	
Snacks	
Goal Met: Yes No	Total Calories:

Date: | Weight:

Include Food and Drink Here | Note Calories Here

Breakfast

Lunch

Dinner

Snacks

Goal Met: Yes   No | Total Calories:

Date:	Weight:
Include Food and Drink Here	Note Calories Here
Breakfast	
Lunch	
Dinner	
Snacks	
Goal Met: Yes No	Total Calories:

Date: | Weight:

Include Food and Drink Here | Note Calories Here

Breakfast

Lunch

Dinner

Snacks

Goal Met: Yes   No | Total Calories:

Date: | Weight:

Include Food and Drink Here | Note Calories Here

Breakfast

Lunch

Dinner

Snacks

Goal Met: Yes   No | Total Calories:

Date:	Weight:
Include Food and Drink Here	Note Calories Here
Breakfast	
Lunch	
Dinner	
Snacks	
Goal Met: Yes No	Total Calories:

Date:	Weight:
Include Food and Drink Here	Note Calories Here
Breakfast	
Lunch	
Dinner	
Snacks	
Goal Met: Yes No	Total Calories:

Date:	Weight:
Include Food and Drink Here	Note Calories Here
Breakfast	
Lunch	
Dinner	
Snacks	
Goal Met: Yes No	Total Calories:

Date: | Weight:

Include Food and Drink Here | Note Calories Here

Breakfast

Lunch

Dinner

Snacks

Goal Met: Yes   No | Total Calories:

Date:	Weight:
Include Food and Drink Here	Note Calories Here
Breakfast	
Lunch	
Dinner	
Snacks	
Goal Met: Yes No	Total Calories:

Date: | Weight:

Include Food and Drink Here | Note Calories Here

Breakfast

Lunch

Dinner

Snacks

Goal Met: Yes   No | Total Calories:

Date:	Weight:
Include Food and Drink Here	Note Calories Here
Breakfast	
Lunch	
Dinner	
Snacks	
Goal Met: Yes No	Total Calories:

Date: | Weight:

Include Food and Drink Here | Note Calories Here

Breakfast

Lunch

Dinner

Snacks

Goal Met: Yes   No | Total Calories:

Date: | Weight:

Include Food and Drink Here | Note Calories Here

Breakfast

_____ | _____
_____ | _____
_____ | _____

Lunch

_____ | _____
_____ | _____
_____ | _____

Dinner

_____ | _____
_____ | _____
_____ | _____

Snacks

_____ | _____
_____ | _____
_____ | _____

Goal Met: Yes   No | Total Calories:

www.ingramcontent.com/pod-product-compliance
Lightning Source LLC
Chambersburg PA
CBHW070643290526
45790CB00001B/173